Family Medical Charts

By Cathy Coulter

Other Books Written by Cathy Coulter

The Man in Red

A Child's Book of Poems

The Little Net Book: Blue

The Little Net Book: Pink

The Little Net Book: Yellow

The Little Net Book: Black

Journal: Lion

Journal: Eye of the Tiger

Whatever: Explore the Possibilities

Books Written under the name of Catherine Coulter

Land Research Records

Census Research Record

My Family Research Plan

Military Research Records

Web Log and Web Accounts

Immigration Research Records

Court House Research Records

Family Group Research Record

Naturalization Research Records

My Family Tree Research Record

My Family Tree Research Notebook

Cemetery and Funeral Home Research Records

My Blood Pressure Chart

Internet Addresses and Accounts

Illness Charts

Doctor_____Phone_____

Doctor_____Phone_____

Hospittal_____Phone_____

Pharmacy_____Phone_____

Emergency Contact_____Phone_____

Emergency Contact_____Phone_____

Emergency Contact_____Phone_____

Medication, Food, Other Items Necessary in Caring for Illness

Over the counter Medications	Foods	Other Items

Medications taking on regular bases

Be sure to use pencil so you can make changes if needed

Name _____

Medication	Dosage	For	Date Started

Name _____

Medication	Dosage	For	Date Started

Medications taking on regular bases

Be sure to use pencil so you can make changes if needed

Name _____

Medication	Dosage	For	Date Started

Name _____

Medication	Dosage	For	Date Started

Surgeries / Procedures

Name _____

What Kind of Surgery	Doctor	For	Date Of

Name _____

What Kind of Surgery	Doctor	For	Date Of

Surgeries / Procedures

Name _____

What Kind of Surgery	Doctor	For	Date Of

Name _____

What Kind of Surgery	Doctor	For	Date Of

ILLNESS CHART

Who_____

Symptoms: ☐ Fever ☐ Cough ☐ Runny nose

☐ Sore Throat ☐ Chills ☐ Vomiting

☐ Diarrhea ☐ Exhaustion

NOTES:

On Set Date_____

Doctor Apt/Rx_____

_____

TEMP	TIME // DAY	MEDS / NOTES:

ILLNESS CHART

Who_____

Symptoms: ☐ Fever ☐ Cough ☐ Runny nose
☐ Sore Throat ☐ Chills ☐ Vomiting
☐ Diarrhea ☐ Exhaustion
NOTES:

On Set Date_____
Doctor Apt/Rx_____

_____

TEMP	TIME // DAY	MEDS / NOTES:

ILLNESS CHART

Who_____

Symptoms: ☐ Fever ☐ Cough ☐ Runny nose
☐ Sore Throat ☐ Chills ☐ Vomiting
☐ Diarrhea ☐ Exhaustion

NOTES:

On Set Date_____
Doctor Apt/Rx_____

_____

TEMP	TIME // DAY	MEDS / NOTES:

ILLNESS CHART

Who_____

Symptoms: ☐ Fever   ☐ Cough   ☐ Runny nose

☐ Sore Throat   ☐ Chills   ☐ Vomiting

☐ Diarrhea   ☐ Exhaustion

NOTES:

On Set Date_____

Doctor Apt/Rx_____

_____

TEMP	TIME // DAY	MEDS / NOTES:

ILLNESS CHART

Who_____

Symptoms: ☐ Fever ☐ Cough ☐ Runny nose

☐ Sore Throat ☐ Chills ☐ Vomiting

☐ Diarrhea ☐ Exhaustion

NOTES:

On Set Date_____

Doctor Apt/Rx_____

_____

TEMP	TIME // DAY	MEDS / NOTES:

ILLNESS CHART

Who_____

Symptoms: ☐ Fever ☐ Cough ☐ Runny nose
☐ Sore Throat ☐ Chills ☐ Vomiting
☐ Diarrhea ☐ Exhaustion

NOTES:

On Set Date_____
Doctor Apt/Rx_____
_____

TEMP	TIME // DAY	MEDS / NOTES:

ILLNESS CHART

Who_____

Symptoms: ☐ Fever ☐ Cough ☐ Runny nose
☐ Sore Throat ☐ Chills ☐ Vomiting
☐ Diarrhea ☐ Exhaustion

NOTES:

On Set Date_____

Doctor Apt/Rx_____

_____

TEMP	TIME // DAY	MEDS / NOTES:

ILLNESS CHART

Who_____

Symptoms: ☐ Fever ☐ Cough ☐ Runny nose
☐ Sore Throat ☐ Chills ☐ Vomiting
☐ Diarrhea ☐ Exhaustion

NOTES:

On Set Date_____
Doctor Apt/Rx_____
_____

TEMP	TIME // DAY	MEDS / NOTES:

ILLNESS CHART

Who_____

Symptoms: ☐ Fever ☐ Cough ☐ Runny nose

☐ Sore Throat ☐ Chills ☐ Vomiting

☐ Diarrhea ☐ Exhaustion

NOTES:

On Set Date_____

Doctor Apt/Rx_____

_____

TEMP	TIME // DAY	MEDS / NOTES:

ILLNESS CHART

Who_____

Symptoms: ☐ Fever ☐ Cough ☐ Runny nose
☐ Sore Throat ☐ Chills ☐ Vomiting
☐ Diarrhea ☐ Exhaustion

NOTES:

On Set Date_____

Doctor Apt/Rx_____

_____

TEMP	TIME // DAY	MEDS / NOTES:

ILLNESS CHART

Who_____

Symptoms: ☐ Fever ☐ Cough ☐ Runny nose

☐ Sore Throat ☐ Chills ☐ Vomiting

☐ Diarrhea ☐ Exhaustion

NOTES:

On Set Date_____

Doctor Apt/Rx_____

_____

TEMP	TIME // DAY	MEDS / NOTES:

ILLNESS CHART

Who_____

Symptoms: ☐ Fever   ☐ Cough   ☐ Runny nose
☐ Sore Throat   ☐ Chills   ☐ Vomiting
☐ Diarrhea   ☐ Exhaustion

NOTES:

On Set Date_____
Doctor Apt/Rx_____
_____

TEMP	TIME // DAY	MEDS / NOTES:

ILLNESS CHART

Who_____

Symptoms: ☐ Fever ☐ Cough ☐ Runny nose
☐ Sore Throat ☐ Chills ☐ Vomiting
☐ Diarrhea ☐ Exhaustion

NOTES:

On Set Date_____

Doctor Apt/Rx_____

_____

TEMP	TIME // DAY	MEDS / NOTES:

ILLNESS CHART

Who_____

Symptoms: ☐ Fever ☐ Cough ☐ Runny nose

☐ Sore Throat ☐ Chills ☐ Vomiting

☐ Diarrhea ☐ Exhaustion

NOTES:

On Set Date_____

Doctor Apt/Rx_____

_____

TEMP	TIME // DAY	MEDS / NOTES:

ILLNESS CHART

Who_____

Symptoms: ☐ Fever ☐ Cough ☐ Runny nose

☐ Sore Throat ☐ Chills ☐ Vomiting

☐ Diarrhea ☐ Exhaustion

NOTES:

On Set Date_____

Doctor Apt/Rx_____

_____

TEMP	TIME // DAY	MEDS / NOTES:

ILLNESS CHART

Who_____

Symptoms: ☐ Fever ☐ Cough ☐ Runny nose
☐ Sore Throat ☐ Chills ☐ Vomiting
☐ Diarrhea ☐ Exhaustion

NOTES:

On Set Date_____
Doctor Apt/Rx_____
_____

TEMP	TIME // DAY	MEDS / NOTES:

Name_____

Name_____

Name_____

Name_____